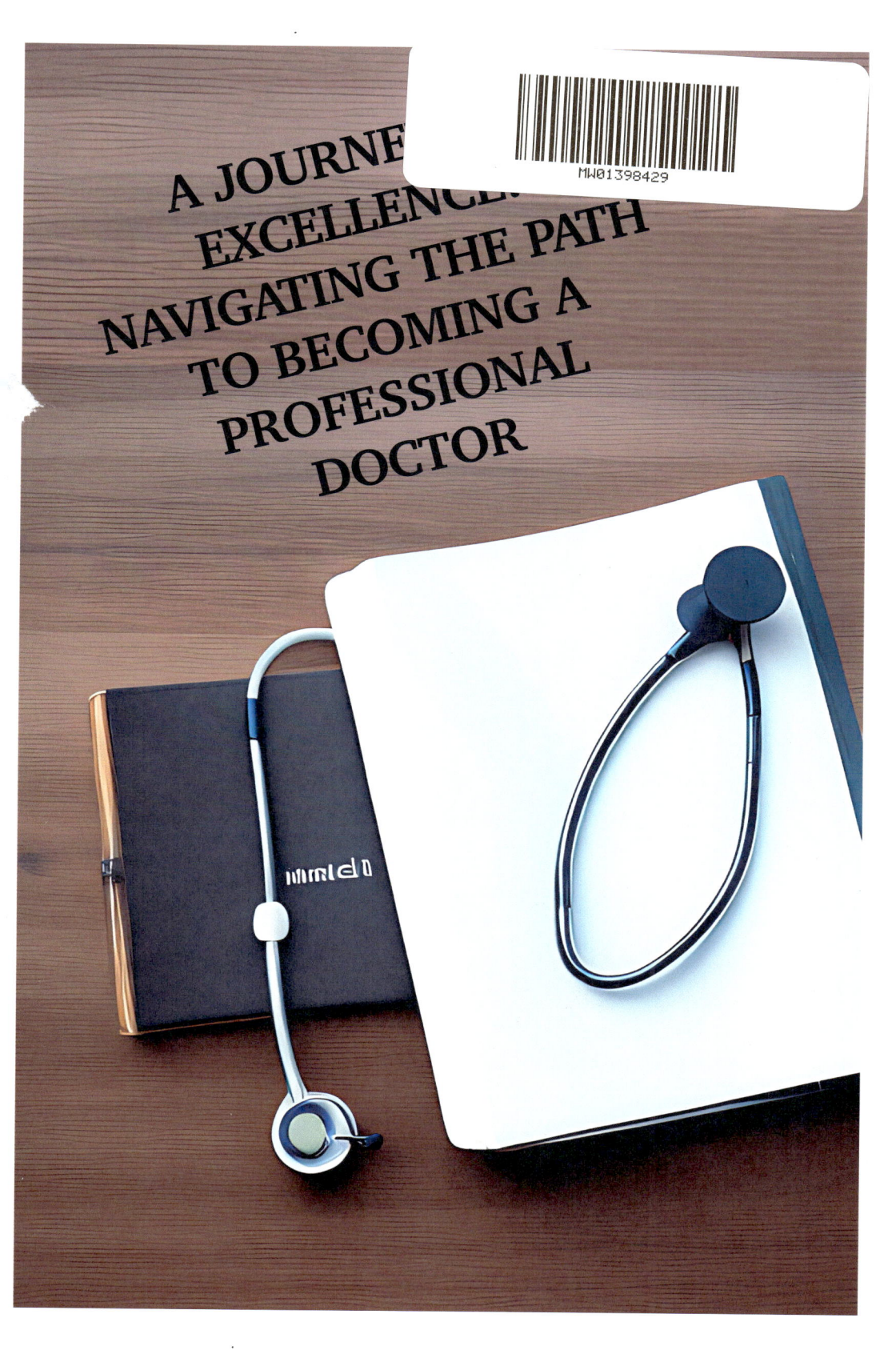

A JOURNEY TO EXCELLENCE: NAVIGATING THE PATH TO BECOMING A PROFESSIONAL DOCTOR

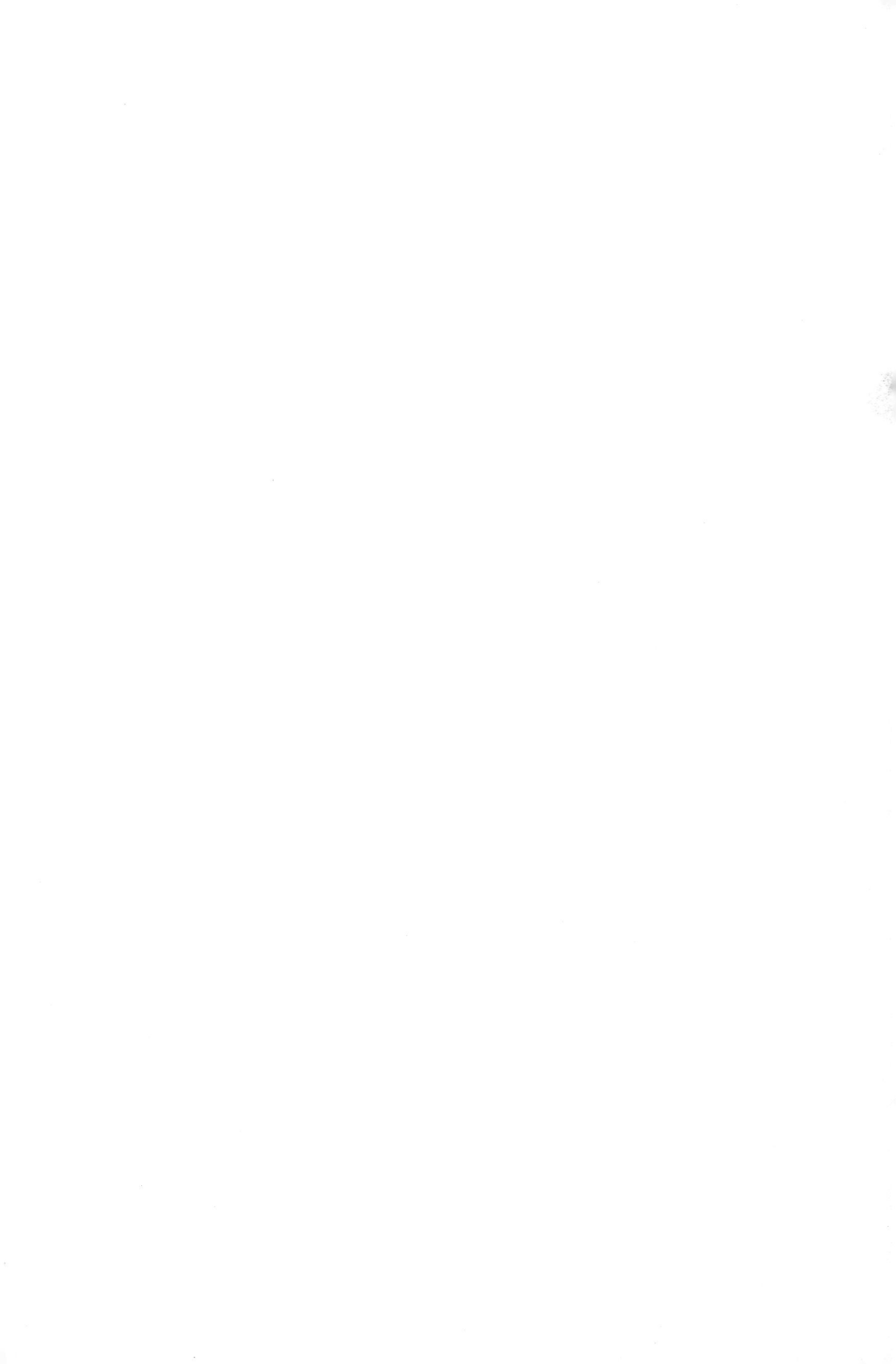

"Ignite the Healing Flame"

Introduction:

Prepare to embark on an extraordinary journey of self-discovery, growth, and transformation. This book is not just a mere collection of information; it is a symphony of inspiration, motivation, and deeply brain-stimulating content that will awaken your senses and ignite a burning desire within you to improve and be less wrong. It is a beacon of light that will guide you towards becoming the best doctor you can possibly be, with an unwavering determination that nothing can extinguish.

In these pages, you will find the keys to unlock your true potential as a medical professional. It is a call to action, urging you to embrace the power of continuous education and self-improvement. Just as dopamine floods our brains with a sense of reward and pleasure, this book will infuse you with an insatiable hunger for knowledge and an unyielding drive to be at the forefront of medical advancements.

Let this book be the catalyst that propels you towards greatness. With each turn of the page, you will be immersed in a world of inspiration and motivation, where the pursuit of excellence becomes your guiding star. As you dive deep into the realms of medical knowledge, empathy, effective communication, and the art of healing, you will realize that nothing can stand in your way. Armed with the wisdom and insights within these chapters, you will become an unstoppable force in the medical field, making a difference in the lives of countless individuals.

So, dear reader, I implore you to take this leap of faith. Open your mind and heart to the possibilities that lie ahead. Let this book be your compass, your guiding light, and your constant companion on this incredible journey towards becoming the best doctor you can be. As long as you keep educating yourself, there will be no limits to what you can achieve. The world awaits your brilliance, and this book will be your trusted ally every step of the way.

"Ignite the Healing Flame"

Content:

- Chapter 1: Exploring the Medical Field
- Understand the different fields of medicine and choose a specialty that aligns with your interests and passion.

- Chapter 2: Undergraduate Education
- Pursue a bachelor's degree, preferably in a science-related field, to meet the prerequisites for medical school. Maintain a strong academic record during this time.

- Chapter 3: Medical School
- Apply and gain acceptance to a medical school. Complete the rigorous coursework, clinical rotations, and exams during the four years of medical school.

- Chapter 4: Residency
- After medical school, you'll need to complete a residency program in your chosen specialty. This can range from three to seven years, depending on the field.

- Chapter 5: Licensure and Board Certification
- Obtain a medical license by passing the required exams in your country or region. Consider pursuing board certification in your specialty for further recognition and credibility.

- Chapter 6: Continuing Education and Professional Development

- Medicine is an ever-evolving field, so it's essential to stay updated with the latest research and advancements. Attend conferences, workshops, and engage in lifelong learning.

- Chapter 7: Building Clinical Experience
- Gain practical experience by working in hospitals, clinics, or other healthcare settings. This will help you refine your skills and build a solid foundation as a doctor.

- Chapter 8: Establishing a Professional Reputation
- Build a network of colleagues, mentors, and fellow healthcare professionals. Contribute to research, publish papers, and participate in professional organizations to enhance your reputation.

"Ignite the Healing Flame"

Chapter 1:

Exploring the Medical Field

The world of medicine is a vast universe filled with endless possibilities. Imagine being able to make a difference in people's lives every day, to provide care and comfort to those in need. As you embark on this journey, take a moment to explore the various fields of medicine. From pediatrics to neurosurgery, from psychiatry to oncology, there is a specialization that awaits your unique set of skills and passions.

Unleashing Your Potential
You have the power within you to become a successful doctor. Your potential knows no bounds, and with each step you take, you are one step closer to realizing your dreams. It may seem daunting at times, but remember that every great doctor started as a novice. Embrace the challenges, learn from your experiences, and never stop striving for excellence. The path ahead may be challenging, but the rewards will be immeasurable.

Nurturing Your Curiosity
In medicine, curiosity is the fuel that propels innovation and progress. As you delve into the intricacies of the human body, let your curiosity guide you. Ask questions, seek answers, and never stop learning. The world of medicine is ever-evolving, and by nurturing your thirst for knowledge, you will always be at the forefront of cutting-edge advancements. Embrace the

joy of discovery and let your curiosity lead you to new horizons.

Embracing Lifelong Learning

Becoming a successful doctor is not just about obtaining a degree; it is a lifelong journey of growth and development. Embrace the concept of lifelong learning, as it will be your compass in navigating the ever-changing landscape of medicine. Attend conferences, engage in research, and collaborate with esteemed colleagues. By embracing continuous education, you will not only enhance your skills but also contribute to the betterment of healthcare.

A Bright Future Awaits

As you embark on this noble path, envision a future filled with endless opportunities. The world needs compassionate, skilled, and dedicated doctors like you. From breakthrough treatments to cutting-edge technologies, the future of medicine holds promises that will revolutionize healthcare. Embrace the possibilities, for your journey has just begun. With each step you take, you are shaping a future where health and well-being thrive, and you have the power to make a lasting impact.

Remember, your journey as a doctor is not just about achieving success, but also about making a difference. Let the joy of helping others and the pursuit of knowledge be your guiding light. Embrace the challenges, nurture your passions, and dare to dream big. Your journey as a doctor is just beginning, and the world eagerly awaits your brilliance and dedication.

"Ignite the Healing Flame"

Chapter 2:

Undergraduate Education

Your journey towards becoming a doctor begins with a solid foundation in undergraduate education. As you embark on this chapter, immerse yourself in a field that ignites your curiosity and passion. Whether it's biology, chemistry, or any other science-related field, choose a major that aligns with your interests. Embrace the joy of learning, absorb knowledge like a sponge, and let your academic record shine brightly. Each step you take in your undergraduate education brings you closer to your dream of healing and making a difference in the world.

Embracing Challenges
The path to becoming a doctor is not without its challenges, but it is these very challenges that shape us into resilient individuals. Embrace the obstacles that come your way, as they are opportunities for growth and self-improvement. Each challenge you overcome, each setback you face, brings you one step closer to becoming the doctor you aspire to be. Remember, it is not about being perfect; it is about being determined and persevering in the face of adversity. Embrace the challenges that come your way, for they will mold you into a stronger and more compassionate healer.

Seeking Mentorship and Guidance
Throughout your journey, seek mentorship and guidance from experienced professionals who have walked the path before you. Their wisdom and insights will not only provide you with invaluable knowledge but

also inspire and uplift you during moments of doubt. Embrace the power of mentorship, for it is through the guidance of others that you can unlock your true potential. Let their experiences and advice deeply stimulate your brain, fueling your desire to improve and be the best version of yourself.

Embracing Diversity
The field of medicine is a tapestry woven with diverse stories, experiences, and perspectives. Embrace the beauty of diversity and open your heart and mind to the richness it brings. Engage with individuals from different backgrounds, cultures, and walks of life. By embracing diversity, you expand your horizons and gain a deeper understanding of humanity. Let the tapestry of diversity inspire you to provide equitable care for all, and be an advocate for those whose voices are often unheard.

A Bright Future Awaits
As you embark on this extraordinary journey, envision a future filled with boundless opportunities. The world of medicine is constantly evolving, offering an abundance of possibilities for growth and contribution. From groundbreaking research to technological advancements, the future holds endless prospects for innovation and improving healthcare. Embrace the bright future that awaits you, for your dedication and passion will create ripples of positive change in the lives of countless individuals. Dream big, aim high, and know that the world eagerly awaits your unique contributions as a doctor.

"Ignite the Healing Flame"

Chapter 3:

The Gateway to Medical School

Congratulations on taking the first step towards your dream of becoming a doctor! Now, it's time to embark on the transformative journey of medical school. As you apply to various institutions, envision yourself walking through the doors of your dream medical school, ready to embrace the challenges and opportunities that lie ahead. The rigorous coursework, clinical rotations, and exams may seem daunting, but remember, each day brings you closer to your ultimate goal. Trust in your abilities, embrace the process, and let the excitement of this chapter deeply stimulate your brain, motivating you to improve and be less wrong.

The Art of Learning

In medical school, the pursuit of knowledge becomes an art form. Embrace the joy of discovery as you dive into the intricacies of human anatomy, physiology, and disease. Each lecture, each patient encounter, and each late-night study session is an opportunity to deepen your understanding and refine your skills. Engage all your senses as you immerse yourself in the world of medicine. Visualize the intricate structures of the human body, listen attentively to the stories of patients, and touch the tools that will become extensions of your healing hands. Let the pursuit of knowledge touch all your senses like dopamine, inspiring you to continuously improve and be the best physician you can be.

The Power of Collaboration

Medicine is not a solitary journey; it is a collaborative endeavor. Throughout your time in medical school, embrace the power of teamwork and collaboration. Engage with your peers, learn from their experiences, and support each other through the ups and downs. Together, you will navigate the challenges and celebrate the victories. Embrace the diverse perspectives and skills that your colleagues bring, for they will expand your horizons and deepen your understanding of patient care. Let the collaborative spirit uplift you, knowing that by working together, you have the power to create an even brighter future for healthcare.

The Patient's Trust

As a future physician, one of the greatest privileges is earning the trust of your patients. Each interaction with a patient is an opportunity to make a profound impact on their lives. Embrace the responsibility that comes with this trust, and let it guide your every action. Listen attentively to their concerns, show empathy and compassion, and always strive to provide the highest quality care. Remember, it is not just the medical knowledge you possess that will heal your patients; it is the human connection, the trust you build, and the genuine care you provide that will make a lasting difference. Let the trust of your patients deeply stimulate your brain, motivating you to continuously improve and be less wrong in your practice.

A Bright Future Awaits

As you near the completion of your medical school journey, envision a future brimming with endless opportunities. The field of medicine is constantly evolving, offering a multitude of paths to explore. From specialized areas of practice to research, teaching, and advocacy, the possibilities are vast. Embrace the bright future that awaits you, knowing that your unique skills and passion will open doors to countless opportunities. Dream big, for your contributions will shape the future of healthcare and positively impact the lives of individuals around the world. Embrace the journey ahead with excitement and anticipation, for the best is yet to come.

"Ignite the Healing Flame"

Chapter 4:

The Path to Specialization

Congratulations on successfully completing medical school! Now, it's time to embark on the next phase of your journey: residency. As you immerse yourself in your chosen specialty, let the knowledge and skills you acquired during medical school come alive. Embrace the challenges and opportunities that lie ahead, for they will deeply stimulate your brain and motivate you to continuously improve and be less wrong in your practice. Each day of residency will be a chance to refine your expertise, honing your abilities to touch all your senses like dopamine.

The Art of Healing

Residency is the crucible where you will develop the art of healing. Embrace the privilege of caring for patients, for each encounter is an opportunity to make a profound impact. As you immerse yourself in the complexity of diagnoses, treatment plans, and surgical procedures, let your mind engage deeply, analyzing every detail with precision. Visualize the intricate workings of the human body, listen attentively to the stories of your patients, and use touch to connect with their physical well-being. This holistic approach to healing will guide you in becoming a compassionate and skilled physician, inspiring you to continuously improve and provide the best possible care.

The Power of Research

Residency offers ample opportunities to engage in research and contribute to the advancement of medicine. Embrace the chance to explore new treatments, technologies, and methodologies. Engage your mind in the pursuit of evidence-based medicine, for it is through research that we can push the boundaries of knowledge and improve patient outcomes. Whether it's in the laboratory, the clinic, or the operating room, let the excitement of discovery deeply stimulate your brain. By engaging in research, you not only contribute to the greater medical community but also open doors to new opportunities and avenues for growth in your career.

Lifelong Learning

As a professional doctor, you are committed to a lifetime of learning. Residency is just the beginning of a journey that will require you to stay up-to-date with the latest advancements in medicine. Embrace the intellectual challenge of staying current in your field, attending conferences, reading research papers, and engaging in continuous education. Let the pursuit of knowledge deeply stimulate your brain, motivating you to continuously improve and be at the forefront of medical breakthroughs. By sharpening your skills and expanding your knowledge, you open doors to countless opportunities for professional growth and impact.

A Bright Future Awaits

As you near the completion of your residency, envision a future brimming with endless possibilities. The world of medicine is vast and ever-evolving, offering a myriad of pathways to explore. From private practice to academic medicine, research, administration, or global health, the opportunities are limitless. Embrace the bright future that awaits you, knowing that your dedication, expertise, and passion will open doors to a fulfilling and impactful career. Dream big, for your contributions have the power to shape the future of healthcare and positively impact the lives of countless individuals. Embrace the journey ahead with excitement and anticipation, for the best is yet to come.

"Ignite the Healing Flame"

Chapter 5:

A Journey of Mastery

Congratulations on embarking on this remarkable journey towards becoming a professional doctor! With each step you take, your path becomes illuminated with the promise of a bright future. Embrace the challenges that lie ahead, for they will deeply stimulate your brain and inspire you to continuously improve. Just as dopamine touches all your senses, the pursuit of mastery in medicine will ignite a fire within you to be the best version of yourself, pushing you to reach new heights of excellence.

Embracing the Complexity

Medicine is a realm of infinite complexity, where every patient presents a unique puzzle waiting to be solved. As you engage your mind in the intricacies of diagnoses, treatments, and therapies, let the vast array of opportunities deeply stimulate your brain. Embrace the joy of unraveling the mysteries of the human body, of understanding its intricate systems and functions. With each case you encounter, your mind will be engaged in a fascinating dance of analysis and problem-solving, propelling you towards continuous improvement and a deeper understanding of the art and science of healing.

The Power of Collaboration

In the world of medicine, collaboration is key. As you progress towards becoming a professional doctor, you will have the privilege of working alongside brilliant minds from various specialties. Together, you will form a network of knowledge and expertise, supporting and inspiring one another to achieve greatness. Let the power of collaboration deeply stimulate your brain, for it is through shared experiences, ideas, and perspectives that we can collectively advance the field of medicine. The opportunities for growth and learning are boundless, and the connections you forge will guide you towards a fulfilling and successful career.

Making a Difference

Each day as a professional doctor offers the opportunity to make a profound difference in the lives of your patients. Let the potential for impact deeply stimulate your brain, inspiring you to continuously improve and be less wrong in your practice. From diagnosing diseases to prescribing treatments, your decisions hold the power to heal, comfort, and transform lives. Embrace the privilege of being a trusted guide on your patients' healing journeys, and let the knowledge that your expertise can bring hope and relief to those in need be a constant source of inspiration.

A World of Possibilities

As you embark on this path towards becoming a professional doctor, a world of endless possibilities unfurls before you. From clinical practice to academia, research, public health, and beyond, the opportunities for growth and impact are vast. Let the vision of a bright future deeply stimulate your brain, igniting a passion within you to explore and embrace the many avenues that lie ahead. With each opportunity you seize, you will continue to evolve, improve, and contribute to the ever-advancing field of medicine. Embrace the journey with excitement and determination, for the world needs your expertise and compassionate care.

"Ignite the Healing Flame"

Chapter 6:

The Art of Lifelong Learning

In the realm of medicine, knowledge is a never-ending journey. As you embark on your path towards becoming a professional doctor, embrace the exhilarating adventure of lifelong learning. Just as dopamine ignites a fire within us to improve and be less wrong, let the pursuit of knowledge deeply stimulate your brain and touch all your senses. Attend conferences, workshops, and immerse yourself in the latest research and advancements. By continuously expanding your understanding and skills, you open doors to a bright future filled with abundant opportunities to make a profound impact.

Embracing the Power of Resilience

In the pursuit of a career as a professional doctor, resilience becomes your steadfast companion. Engage your mind with the understanding that challenges will arise, but they are the catalysts for growth and improvement. Embrace the art of resilience and let it deeply stimulate your brain, for it is through overcoming obstacles that we become stronger and more capable. With each setback, remember that a brighter future awaits, filled with countless chances to rise above and make a lasting difference in the lives of others.

The Healing Power of Compassion

As a professional doctor, you possess a unique ability to touch the lives of others with compassion and care. Let the immense power of empathy deeply stimulate your brain, for it is through understanding and connecting with your patients on a profound level that healing truly begins. Engage your mind in the art of compassionate care, for it is this quality that uplifts and inspires both you and your patients. As you navigate the complexities of medicine, never underestimate the transformative impact a kind word, a gentle touch, or a listening ear can have on someone's journey to recovery.

Embracing a Multidimensional Approach

In the world of medicine, opportunities abound to engage your mind in a multidimensional approach to care. As a professional doctor, you have the privilege to explore diverse fields such as research, public health, and academia. Let the vast array of possibilities deeply stimulate your brain, for it is through embracing these opportunities that you can make an even greater impact. Seize the chance to contribute to groundbreaking research, advocate for healthcare policy changes, or inspire future generations through teaching. The possibilities are endless, and each avenue you explore will further enrich your journey towards a fulfilling and accomplished career.

A Symphony of Collaboration

Medicine is not a solo endeavor, but rather a symphony of collaboration. As a professional doctor, you will work alongside a diverse team of healthcare professionals united in their mission to provide the best possible care. Engage your mind in the power of teamwork, for it is through the collective efforts of many that true progress is made. Let the exhilaration of collaboration deeply stimulate your brain, as you exchange ideas, learn from others, and together, create a harmonious orchestra of healing. Embrace the opportunities to connect and collaborate, for in these partnerships lies the potential for immense growth, fulfillment, and the realization of a bright and prosperous future.

"Ignite the Healing Flame"

Chapter 7:

The Crucial Role of Clinical Experience

In the realm of medicine, clinical experience serves as the anchor upon which we build our expertise. Engage your mind with the understanding that every interaction, every patient encounter, is an opportunity for deep brain stimulation and growth. By immersing yourself in hospitals, clinics, and other healthcare settings, you will embark on a journey of practical experience that will refine your skills and solidify your foundation as a doctor. As you engage in these real-world scenarios, let the sensation of dopamine fill your senses, inspiring you to continuously improve and strive for excellence.

Embracing the Art of Problem-Solving

As a professional doctor, your mind is a powerful instrument, capable of unraveling the mysteries of the human body. Engage your mind in the art of problem-solving, for it is through this process that you will uncover innovative solutions and pave the way for brighter futures. Let the thrill of deeply stimulating your brain with complex medical cases guide you towards a bright future filled with opportunities to showcase your analytical skills. As you navigate the intricate web of symptoms, diagnoses, and treatment plans, remember that each challenge presents a chance to be less wrong and inspire others with your relentless pursuit of knowledge.

The Symphony of Continuity in Care

In the world of medicine, the continuity of care is a symphony in which you play a pivotal role. Engage your mind in the interconnectedness of healthcare, for it is through this collaboration that we create a brighter future for our patients. Let the sensation of dopamine fill your senses as you deeply stimulate your brain with the understanding that your actions can have a profound impact on someone's life. From diagnosis to treatment, from follow-up visits to long-term care, embrace the opportunities to build lasting relationships and provide comprehensive care. Each moment spent engaging in the continuum of care is a chance to uplift, inspire, and make a lasting difference.

Embracing the Art of Communication

As a professional doctor, your ability to communicate effectively is paramount. Engage your mind in the art of compassionate communication, for it is through these interactions that you will touch the lives of your patients and inspire hope. Let the sensation of dopamine fill your senses as you deeply stimulate your brain with the understanding that your words and gestures can have a profound impact. Whether it's breaking difficult news with empathy, translating complex medical jargon into understandable terms, or simply lending a listening ear, each communication opportunity is a chance to uplift, inspire, and forge connections that will guide your patients towards a brighter future.

Embracing the Limitless Possibilities

As a professional doctor, the future is ablaze with limitless possibilities. Engage your mind in the vast array of opportunities that lie ahead, for it is through this exploration that you will find your own unique path to success. Let the sensation of dopamine fill your senses as you deeply stimulate your brain, for the journey towards becoming a doctor is just the beginning. From specializing in a specific field to becoming a leader in healthcare administration, from conducting groundbreaking research to advocating for healthcare policy changes, the opportunities to shape a brighter future are endless. Embrace the path less traveled, dare to dream big, and let the fire of passion and possibility guide you towards a professional career filled with inspiration, fulfillment, and the relentless pursuit of excellence.

"Ignite the Healing Flame"

Chapter 8:

Nurturing the Seeds of Professional Growth

In the vast expanse of the medical universe, the journey towards becoming a professional doctor begins with the cultivation of a stellar reputation. Engage your mind with the understanding that building a network of colleagues, mentors, and fellow healthcare professionals is the celestial path towards success. Let the sensation of dopamine fill your senses as you deeply stimulate your brain, for each connection forged is a constellation of opportunities, guiding you towards a future brimming with possibilities. Embrace the power of these relationships, for they will uplift, inspire, and propel you towards the stars, where your brilliance as a professional doctor will illuminate the world.

Illuminating the Path of Scientific Discovery

As a professional doctor, your quest for knowledge is not limited to the confines of patient care. Engage your mind in the pursuit of scientific enlightenment, for it is through research, papers, and groundbreaking discoveries that you leave an indelible mark on the medical landscape. Let the sensation of dopamine fill your senses as you deeply stimulate your brain, for each contribution to the realm of scientific inquiry ignites a celestial fire within, inspiring you to reach greater heights. Embrace the opportunity to unravel the mysteries of medicine, to challenge the boundaries of what is known, and to shape a future where health and healing are illuminated by your brilliance.

The Symphony of Professional Organizations

In the symphony of healthcare, professional organizations compose the harmonious notes that orchestrate our collective advancement. Engage your mind with the understanding that by participating in these organizations, you join a celestial ensemble, where opportunities to learn, connect, and grow abound. Let the sensation of dopamine fill your senses as you deeply stimulate your brain, for each involvement in these celestial gatherings is a chance to expand your horizons, exchange ideas, and be surrounded by the brightest minds in the field. Embrace the power of these organizations, for they will uplift, inspire, and guide you towards a professional future resounding with success and fulfillment.

The Cosmos of Lifelong Learning

As a professional doctor, the quest for knowledge knows no bounds. Engage your mind in the realization that the pursuit of learning is an eternal voyage, where each discovery takes you closer to the celestial pinnacle of expertise. Let the sensation of dopamine fill your senses as you deeply stimulate your brain, for every new skill acquired, every piece of knowledge assimilated, propels you towards excellence. Embrace the galaxies of opportunities to engage in continuing education, to attend conferences, and to immerse yourself in the ever-evolving cosmos of medical knowledge. By embracing this thirst for lifelong learning, you will inspire others, improve your practice, and journey towards a future where your brilliance as a professional doctor shines like a supernova.

The Constellations of Purpose and Fulfillment

In the vastness of the medical universe, the pursuit of becoming a professional doctor is not merely a dream, but a calling that resonates deep within your soul. Engage your mind with the understanding that your journey towards this noble profession is a celestial alignment of purpose and fulfillment. Let the sensation of dopamine fill your senses as you deeply stimulate your brain, for the realization of your dreams will bring unparalleled joy and satisfaction. Embrace the knowledge that by embarking on this path, you have the power to heal, to comfort, and to make a lasting impact on the lives of countless individuals. As you close this chapter and embark on your journey towards becoming a professional doctor, remember that the universe is waiting for your brilliance to shine, for your passion to illuminate, and for your dedication to inspire. The cosmos of opportunities awaits, and the stars align in your favor.

"Ignite the Healing Flame"

Note to self:

Remember, becoming a successful doctor requires not only academic excellence but also empathy, effective communication skills, and a genuine desire to help others. This brief overview should give you a starting point, but I encourage you to conduct further research and seek guidance from professionals in the medical field to get more in-depth information.

"Ignite the Healing Flame"

We would appreciate your feedback:

"If you liked this book, then I need your help! Your feedback is invaluable in shaping future books and topics that resonate with readers like you. It not only gives me a better understanding of what you want to read about, but it also helps my book gain more visibility in a crowded market. Taking just a minute of your time to leave an honest review would mean the world to me.

Your review can make a significant impact, allowing others to discover and benefit from the empowering words within these pages. Your support will help spread the message of unstoppable potential and inspire others to overcome any obstacle in their path. Remember, you are unstoppable, and your feedback is a powerful tool to make a difference.

Please consider leaving a review on platforms like Amazon, Goodreads, or any other preferred book review site. Your thoughts and opinions matter greatly, and I genuinely appreciate your support.

For updates, inspirations, and more, follow us on social media @ [insert social media handle]. Together, let's continue to spread the message of empowerment and love. You are incredible, and I am grateful to have you as part of this journey. Thank you!

ABOUT THE AUTHOR

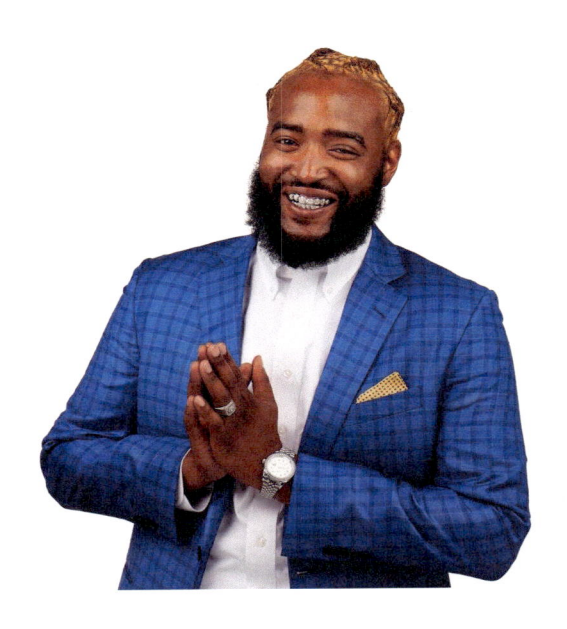

As the author of a best-selling book company, I understand the importance of providing guidance and inspiration to those who are on a journey of self-discovery and personal growth. I know what it feels like to be held back and hindered by self-doubt and uncertainty, and I am determined to do the total opposite.

My books are meticulously crafted to touch all your senses, to deeply stimulate your mind, and to ignite that spark of inspiration within you. I want to create an experience that goes beyond just reading words on a page, but rather transports you to a world where anything is possible and where you are empowered to take charge of your own destiny.

Through engaging storytelling, practical exercises, and thought-provoking insights, my books will guide you on a transformative journey. They will challenge you to break free from limiting beliefs, embrace your true potential, and navigate the obstacles that stand in your way.

So, if you are in search of a book that will truly make a difference in your life, look no further. Join me on this incredible adventure and let my words become the catalyst for your personal and professional success. Together, we will overcome challenges, embrace growth, and unlock the extraordinary possibilities that await you.

Made in the USA
Columbia, SC
11 May 2025